30-MINUTE RENAL DIETS COOKBOOK

Quick & Delicious: Discover Easy Recipes For Kidney Wellness, Perfect For Busty Lifestyles, Boost Kidney Health With Every Bite

Elizabeth Francis

Table of Contents

CHAPTER ONE 4
    Understanding the Renal Diet 4
    What is the Renal Diet? 4
    Why is it Important? 5
    Guidelines and Restrictions 6

CHAPTER TWO 10
    Quick and Easy Breakfast Recipes 10
    Low-Potassium Pancakes 10
    High-Protein Smoothies 12

CHAPTER THREE 16
    Simple Lunch Ideas for Renal Health 16
    Tuna Salad with Kidney-Friendly Ingredients 16
    Vegetable Stir-Fry with Low-Sodium Sauce 18
    Quinoa and Black Bean Salad 19

CHAPTER FOUR 22
    Delicious Dinners in 30 Minutes or Less 22

CHAPTER FIVE 28
    Snacks and Appetizers for Renal-Friendly Eating 28

CHAPTER SIX 33
    Desserts without Compromising Kidney Health 33

Homemade Electrolyte Drinks..40

CHAPTER EIGHT..42

Renal-Friendly Meal Prep Tips and Tricks 42

Proper Storage of Kidney-Safe Ingredients 43

Planning Balanced Meals in Advance 44

CHAPTER NINE 46

Dining Out and Managing the Renal Diet 46

How to Navigate Restaurant Menus 46

Tips for Making Special Requests 47

Identifying Hidden Sodium and Potassium 48

CHAPTER TEN 51

Staying Motivated and Adapting to the Renal Diet.................51

Setting Realistic Goals..51

Celebrating Small Victories 52

Finding Support and Resources 53

CHAPTER ELEVEN 55

RENAL DIETS AND THEIR PREPARATION 55

THE END 105

COPYRIGHT © 2023

All rights reserved. No part of this publication may be reproduced, distributed, or transmitted in any form or by any means, including photocopying, recording, or other electronic or mechanical methods, without the prior written permission of the publisher, except in the case of brief quotations embodied in critical reviews and certain other noncommercial uses permitted by copyright law.

CHAPTER ONE

Understanding the Renal Diet

What is the Renal Diet?

The renal diet, also known as the kidney diet, is a dietary plan specifically tailored for individuals with kidney disease or other kidney-related conditions. It emphasizes controlling certain nutrients to prevent the buildup of waste products and fluid in the body, which the kidneys may struggle to filter efficiently. Essentially, the renal diet aims to lessen the workload on the kidneys and maintain overall health.

One of the primary functions of the kidneys is to filter waste and excess fluids from the bloodstream, excreting them as urine. However, when kidney function is compromised, these waste products can accumulate in the body, leading to various complications such as high blood pressure, fluid retention, and electrolyte imbalances. The renal diet helps manage these issues by regulating the intake of certain nutrients that the kidneys have difficulty processing.

The key components of the renal diet include controlling the intake of protein, sodium, potassium, phosphorus, and fluids. These nutrients play crucial roles in maintaining overall health, but individuals with kidney disease need to be mindful of their consumption to prevent further kidney damage and manage symptoms effectively.

Why is it Important?

The importance of the renal diet cannot be overstated for individuals with kidney disease. Proper nutrition plays a critical role in managing the progression of kidney disease, alleviating symptoms, and improving overall quality of life.

1. **Managing Kidney Function**: The renal diet is designed to reduce the workload on the kidneys by controlling the intake of certain nutrients. By limiting the consumption of protein, sodium, potassium, phosphorus, and fluids, individuals with kidney disease can help slow down the decline in kidney function and delay the need for dialysis or kidney transplantation.

2. **Preventing Complications**: Kidney disease can lead to various complications such as high blood pressure, fluid retention, electrolyte imbalances, and bone disorders. By following a renal diet, individuals can minimize the risk of these complications and improve their overall health outcomes.

3. **Controlling Symptoms**: Many individuals with kidney disease experience symptoms such as fatigue, nausea, loss of appetite, and swelling. The renal diet can help alleviate these

symptoms by providing a well-balanced and nutrient-rich eating plan that supports overall health and well-being.

4. **Improving Quality of Life**: Adhering to a renal diet can significantly improve the quality of life for individuals with kidney disease. By managing symptoms, preventing complications, and slowing down the progression of the disease, individuals can enjoy a better quality of life and engage in activities they enjoy with greater ease.

5. **Customized Approach**: The renal diet is not a one-size-fits-all approach; it is tailored to individual needs based on the stage of kidney disease, overall health status, and other factors. This personalized approach ensures that individuals receive the appropriate level of nutrient restriction and support to effectively manage their condition.

Guidelines and Restrictions

Adhering to the renal diet involves following specific guidelines and restrictions to control the intake of certain nutrients. While the exact recommendations may vary depending on individual circumstances, there are some general guidelines that apply to most individuals with kidney disease.

1. **Protein Restriction**: Protein is essential for building and repairing tissues, but excessive protein intake can put strain on the kidneys. Therefore, individuals with kidney disease are often advised to limit their protein intake, especially if

their kidney function is significantly impaired. High-quality protein sources such as lean meats, poultry, fish, eggs, and dairy products may be included in moderation, while high-protein foods such as red meat, processed meats, and certain dairy products should be limited.

2. **Sodium Restriction**: Sodium, found in salt and many processed foods, can contribute to fluid retention and high blood pressure, both of which are common complications of kidney disease. Therefore, individuals are typically advised to limit their sodium intake to help control fluid balance and blood pressure. This may involve reducing the use of table salt, avoiding high-sodium processed foods, and choosing fresh or minimally processed foods whenever possible.

3. **Potassium Restriction**: Potassium is a mineral that plays a vital role in nerve and muscle function, but excessive potassium levels can be dangerous for individuals with kidney disease, especially if their kidneys are unable to excrete it efficiently. Therefore, potassium intake may need to be restricted, particularly for individuals with advanced kidney disease. Foods high in potassium, such as bananas, oranges, tomatoes, potatoes, and certain other fruits and vegetables, may need to be limited or avoided.

4. **Phosphorus Restriction**: Phosphorus is a mineral that works closely with calcium to build and maintain healthy bones and

teeth. However, elevated phosphorus levels are common in individuals with kidney disease and can contribute to bone disorders and cardiovascular complications. Therefore, phosphorus intake may need to be restricted, and individuals may need to avoid high-phosphorus foods such as dairy products, nuts, seeds, whole grains, and processed foods containing phosphate additives.

5. **Fluid Restriction**: Individuals with kidney disease may experience fluid retention and swelling due to impaired kidney function. Therefore, they may need to restrict their fluid intake to help manage these symptoms and prevent complications such as high blood pressure and fluid overload. The exact fluid restriction may vary depending on individual circumstances, but healthcare providers typically provide guidance on how much fluid is safe for each individual.

In addition to these specific guidelines, individuals with kidney disease are encouraged to follow a well-balanced diet that includes a variety of nutrient-rich foods such as fruits, vegetables, whole grains, and healthy fats. Portion control, meal planning, and regular monitoring of nutritional status are also important aspects of managing the renal diet effectively. Consulting with a registered dietitian or healthcare provider who specializes in kidney disease can provide personalized guidance and support to help individuals navigate the complexities of the renal diet and optimize their nutritional health.

CHAPTER TWO

Quick and Easy Breakfast Recipes

Breakfast is often hailed as the most important meal of the day, yet it's also the one many people struggle to find time for. However, with a little planning and creativity, it's possible to whip up nutritious and delicious breakfasts in no time. Here are some quick and easy breakfast recipes to start your day off right.

Low-Potassium Pancakes

Pancakes are a classic breakfast option loved by many. However, traditional pancake recipes can be high in potassium, which may not be suitable for individuals with kidney disease or those following a low-potassium diet. Here's a simple recipe for low-potassium pancakes that are both tasty and kidney-friendly.

Ingredients:

- 1 cup all-purpose flour
- 1 tablespoon sugar
- 1 teaspoon baking powder
- 1/2 teaspoon baking soda
- 1/4 teaspoon salt
- 1 cup buttermilk (or substitute with a mixture of milk and lemon juice)

- 1 large egg
- 2 tablespoons unsalted butter, melted
- Cooking spray or additional butter for greasing the pan

Instructions:

1. In a large mixing bowl, combine the flour, sugar, baking powder, baking soda, and salt. Mix well to ensure even distribution of the dry ingredients.

2. In a separate bowl, whisk together the buttermilk, egg, and melted butter until smooth.

3. Pour the wet ingredients into the dry ingredients and stir until just combined. Be careful not to overmix; a few lumps are okay.

4. Heat a non-stick skillet or griddle over medium heat and lightly coat it with cooking spray or butter.

5. Pour about 1/4 cup of batter onto the hot skillet for each pancake. Cook until bubbles form on the surface and the edges start to look set, then flip and cook for an additional 1-2 minutes until golden brown.

6. Repeat with the remaining batter, greasing the skillet as needed between batches.

7. Serve the pancakes warm with your choice of toppings such as fresh berries, sliced bananas, a drizzle of honey, or a dollop of Greek yogurt.

These low-potassium pancakes are a satisfying and kidney-friendly breakfast option that's quick and easy to prepare. They're sure to become a favorite among your family and friends, whether or not they have specific dietary restrictions.

High-Protein Smoothies

Smoothies are a fantastic breakfast option for busy mornings, as they can be prepared in minutes and customized to suit your taste preferences and nutritional needs. This recipe for high-protein smoothies is perfect for fueling your day and keeping you satisfied until your next meal.

Ingredients:

- 1 cup unsweetened almond milk (or any milk of your choice)
- 1/2 cup plain Greek yogurt
- 1 scoop of your favorite protein powder (such as whey, soy, or pea protein)
- 1/2 ripe banana, frozen
- 1/2 cup frozen mixed berries (such as strawberries, blueberries, and raspberries)
- 1 tablespoon almond butter or peanut butter

- Optional: honey or maple syrup for sweetness, spinach or kale for added nutrients

Instructions:

1. In a blender, combine the almond milk, Greek yogurt, protein powder, frozen banana, frozen berries, and almond butter.

2. Blend on high speed until smooth and creamy, adding more almond milk if necessary to reach your desired consistency.

3. Taste the smoothie and adjust the sweetness if needed by adding a drizzle of honey or maple syrup.

4. For an extra nutritional boost, you can add a handful of spinach or kale to the blender and blend until smooth.

5. Pour the smoothie into a glass and enjoy immediately, or pour it into a portable container to take on the go.

These high-protein smoothies are a convenient and delicious breakfast option that's packed with nutrients to keep you energized throughout the morning. Feel free to experiment with different fruit combinations and add-ins to create your perfect smoothie blend.

Egg White Omelette Variations

Egg white omelettes are a fantastic low-calorie, high-protein breakfast option that can be customized with a variety of fillings to suit your taste preferences. Here are three delicious variations to try:

Mediterranean Omelette:

- Ingredients: Egg whites, diced tomatoes, chopped spinach, sliced olives, crumbled feta cheese, fresh basil, salt, and pepper.

- Instructions: Whisk together the egg whites and pour them into a heated non-stick skillet. Sprinkle the tomatoes, spinach, olives, and feta cheese over one half of the omelette. Cook until the edges are set, then fold the omelette in half and continue cooking until the cheese is melted and the omelette is cooked through. Garnish with fresh basil and season with salt and pepper to taste.

Western Omelette:

- Ingredients: Egg whites, diced bell peppers, diced onions, diced ham or turkey, shredded cheddar cheese, salt, and pepper.

- Instructions: Whisk together the egg whites and pour them into a heated non-stick skillet. Sprinkle the bell peppers, onions, and ham or turkey over one half of the omelette. Cook until the edges are set, then sprinkle the shredded cheddar cheese over the fillings. Fold the omelette in half and continue cooking until the cheese is melted and the omelette is cooked through. Season with salt and pepper to taste.

Vegetarian Omelette:

- Ingredients: Egg whites, sliced mushrooms, diced bell peppers, diced onions, chopped spinach, shredded mozzarella cheese, salt, and pepper.

- Instructions: Whisk together the egg whites and pour them into a heated non-stick skillet. Sprinkle the mushrooms, bell peppers, onions, and spinach over one half of the omelette. Cook until the edges are set, then sprinkle the shredded mozzarella cheese over the fillings. Fold the omelette in half and continue cooking until the cheese is melted and the omelette is cooked through. Season with salt and pepper to taste.

These egg white omelette variations are quick and easy to prepare, making them perfect for busy weekday mornings. Feel free to customize the fillings based on your preferences and dietary restrictions, and enjoy a nutritious and satisfying breakfast to kickstart your day.

CHAPTER THREE

Simple Lunch Ideas for Renal Health

When it comes to maintaining renal health, a well-balanced diet plays a crucial role. Lunchtime offers an opportunity to fuel your body with nutritious foods that support kidney function while satisfying your taste buds. Here are three simple lunch ideas specifically designed to promote renal health.

Tuna Salad with Kidney-Friendly Ingredients

Tuna salad is a versatile and protein-rich dish that can be easily customized to fit a renal diet. By incorporating kidney-friendly ingredients and limiting sodium, you can create a delicious and nourishing lunch option.

Ingredients:

- Canned tuna in water, drained
- Chopped celery
- Chopped red bell pepper
- Chopped cucumber
- Chopped red onion
- Low-sodium mayonnaise or Greek yogurt
- Dijon mustard

- Lemon juice
- Salt-free seasoning blend (such as Mrs. Dash)
- Fresh parsley or dill, chopped (optional)
- Whole grain bread or lettuce leaves for serving

Instructions:

1. In a mixing bowl, combine the drained tuna, chopped celery, red bell pepper, cucumber, and red onion.

2. In a separate small bowl, whisk together the low-sodium mayonnaise or Greek yogurt, Dijon mustard, lemon juice, and salt-free seasoning blend until smooth and well combined.

3. Pour the dressing over the tuna and vegetable mixture and toss until everything is evenly coated.

4. Taste the salad and adjust the seasoning as needed, adding more lemon juice or seasoning blend if desired.

5. If desired, sprinkle fresh parsley or dill over the salad for added flavor and freshness.

6. Serve the tuna salad on whole grain bread for a classic sandwich, or scoop it onto lettuce leaves for a lighter, low-carb option.

This tuna salad is packed with protein and kidney-friendly nutrients, making it an excellent choice for individuals with renal health concerns. Feel free to customize the recipe with your favorite vegetables and seasonings to suit your taste preferences.

Vegetable Stir-Fry with Low-Sodium Sauce

Stir-fries are a quick and convenient way to incorporate a variety of vegetables into your diet while keeping sodium levels in check. By using a low-sodium sauce and lean protein, you can enjoy a flavorful and kidney-friendly lunch that's both satisfying and nutritious.

Ingredients:

- Assorted vegetables (such as bell peppers, broccoli, carrots, snap peas, and mushrooms), sliced or chopped
- Lean protein of your choice (such as chicken breast, tofu, or shrimp), sliced or cubed
- Low-sodium stir-fry sauce (store-bought or homemade)
- Cooked brown rice or quinoa for serving

Instructions:

1. Heat a large skillet or wok over medium-high heat and add a small amount of oil.
2. Add the sliced or chopped vegetables to the skillet and stir-fry for a few minutes until they start to soften slightly.

3. Push the vegetables to one side of the skillet and add the lean protein to the empty side. Cook until the protein is cooked through and lightly browned.

4. Combine the vegetables and protein in the skillet and pour the low-sodium stir-fry sauce over the mixture. Stir well to coat everything evenly.

5. Continue cooking for a few more minutes until the sauce is heated through and the vegetables are tender-crisp.

6. Serve the vegetable stir-fry over cooked brown rice or quinoa for a complete and satisfying meal.

This vegetable stir-fry is loaded with fiber, vitamins, and minerals, making it an excellent choice for promoting renal health. The low-sodium sauce adds flavor without compromising on kidney-friendly nutrition, making this lunch option both delicious and nourishing.

Quinoa and Black Bean Salad

Quinoa and black bean salad is a nutrient-dense and protein-packed dish that's perfect for a renal-friendly lunch. By incorporating whole grains, legumes, and fresh vegetables, you can create a satisfying and balanced meal that supports kidney health.

Ingredients:

- Cooked quinoa
- Cooked black beans (canned or homemade), drained and rinsed
- Diced tomatoes
- Diced bell peppers (any color)
- Diced red onion
- Chopped cilantro
- Lime juice
- Extra-virgin olive oil
- Salt-free seasoning blend
- Avocado slices (optional)

Instructions:

1. In a large mixing bowl, combine the cooked quinoa, black beans, diced tomatoes, bell peppers, red onion, and chopped cilantro.
2. In a small bowl, whisk together the lime juice, extra-virgin olive oil, and salt-free seasoning blend until well combined.
3. Pour the dressing over the quinoa and black bean mixture and toss until everything is evenly coated.

4. Taste the salad and adjust the seasoning as needed, adding more lime juice or seasoning blend if desired.

5. If desired, garnish the salad with slices of avocado for added creaminess and healthy fats.

6. Serve the quinoa and black bean salad as a standalone dish or alongside grilled chicken, fish, or tofu for additional protein.

This quinoa and black bean salad is packed with fiber, protein, and essential nutrients, making it an excellent choice for individuals looking to support their kidney health. It's versatile, satisfying, and bursting with flavor, making it a lunch option you'll want to enjoy again and again.

CHAPTER FOUR

Delicious Dinners in 30 Minutes or Less

Preparing dinner doesn't have to be time-consuming or complicated. With the right recipes and a little bit of planning, you can whip up delicious and nutritious meals in 30 minutes or less. Here are three quick and easy dinner ideas that are sure to satisfy your taste buds without keeping you stuck in the kitchen for hours.

Lemon Herb Baked Fish Fillets

Baked fish fillets are a healthy and flavorful dinner option that can be on the table in 30 minutes or less. This recipe features a zesty lemon herb marinade that adds brightness and depth of flavor to the fish.

Ingredients:

- Fish fillets of your choice (such as tilapia, salmon, or cod)
- Fresh lemon juice
- Olive oil
- Minced garlic
- Chopped fresh herbs (such as parsley, dill, or thyme)
- Salt and pepper

Instructions:

1. Preheat your oven to 375°F (190°C) and lightly grease a baking dish with olive oil or cooking spray.

2. In a small bowl, whisk together the fresh lemon juice, olive oil, minced garlic, chopped herbs, salt, and pepper to create the marinade.

3. Place the fish fillets in the prepared baking dish and pour the marinade over the top, ensuring that the fillets are evenly coated.

4. Bake the fish in the preheated oven for 15-20 minutes, depending on the thickness of the fillets, or until they are cooked through and flake easily with a fork.

5. Remove the fish from the oven and let it rest for a few minutes before serving.

6. Garnish the baked fish fillets with additional fresh herbs and lemon slices, if desired, and serve with your favorite side dishes such as steamed vegetables, rice, or quinoa.

This lemon herb baked fish is light, flavorful, and perfect for a quick and easy weeknight dinner. It's also highly versatile, so feel free to experiment with different types of fish and herbs to suit your taste preferences.

Turkey Meatballs with Zucchini Noodles

Turkey meatballs are a lean and protein-packed alternative to traditional beef meatballs, and when paired with zucchini noodles, they make for a healthy and satisfying dinner option. This recipe comes together quickly and is perfect for busy evenings when you need dinner on the table fast.

Ingredients:

- Ground turkey
- Minced garlic
- Chopped fresh parsley
- Grated Parmesan cheese
- Salt and pepper
- Olive oil
- Zucchini
- Marinara sauce (store-bought or homemade)

Instructions:

1. In a large mixing bowl, combine the ground turkey, minced garlic, chopped parsley, grated Parmesan cheese, salt, and pepper. Use your hands to mix everything together until well combined.
2. Roll the turkey mixture into small meatballs, about 1 inch in diameter, and place them on a plate or baking sheet.

3. Heat a large skillet over medium heat and add a drizzle of olive oil. Once the oil is hot, add the turkey meatballs to the skillet and cook for 8-10 minutes, turning occasionally, until browned on all sides and cooked through.

4. While the meatballs are cooking, use a spiralizer or vegetable peeler to create zucchini noodles (also known as zoodles) from the zucchini.

5. Once the meatballs are cooked, remove them from the skillet and set them aside. Add the zucchini noodles to the skillet and cook for 2-3 minutes, tossing occasionally, until they are just tender.

6. Return the turkey meatballs to the skillet, along with the marinara sauce, and toss everything together until the meatballs and noodles are evenly coated in the sauce.

7. Serve the turkey meatballs and zucchini noodles hot, garnished with additional grated Parmesan cheese and fresh parsley, if desired.

This turkey meatballs with zucchini noodles recipe is a healthy and delicious dinner option that's ready in 30 minutes or less. It's packed with protein, fiber, and flavor, making it a satisfying meal the whole family will love.

Chicken and Vegetable Stir-Fry

Stir-fries are a quick and versatile dinner option that can be customized with your favorite proteins and vegetables. This chicken and vegetable stir-fry comes together in a flash and is perfect for busy weeknights when you need a healthy meal in a hurry.

Ingredients:

- Boneless, skinless chicken breasts or thighs, sliced into thin strips
- Soy sauce (low-sodium if possible)
- Sesame oil
- Minced garlic
- Sliced bell peppers (any color)
- Sliced carrots
- Broccoli florets
- Snow peas
- Cooked brown rice or quinoa for serving

Instructions:

1. In a small bowl, combine the sliced chicken strips with soy sauce, sesame oil, and minced garlic. Toss to coat the chicken evenly in the marinade and set aside to marinate for a few minutes.

2. Heat a large skillet or wok over medium-high heat and add a drizzle of sesame oil. Once the oil is hot, add the marinated chicken strips to the skillet and cook for 5-6 minutes, stirring occasionally, until they are cooked through and lightly browned.

3. Remove the cooked chicken from the skillet and set it aside. Add a bit more sesame oil to the skillet if needed, then add the sliced bell peppers, carrots, broccoli florets, and snow peas.

4. Stir-fry the vegetables for 3-4 minutes until they are tender-crisp and brightly colored.

5. Return the cooked chicken to the skillet and toss everything together until the chicken and vegetables are evenly combined.

6. Serve the chicken and vegetable stir-fry hot, over cooked brown rice or quinoa for a complete and satisfying meal.

CHAPTER FIVE

Snacks and Appetizers for Renal-Friendly Eating

Maintaining a renal-friendly diet involves making thoughtful choices about the foods you eat throughout the day, including snacks and appetizers. By selecting nutrient-dense options that are low in sodium, potassium, and phosphorus, you can support your kidney health while satisfying your cravings between meals. Here are three delicious snack and appetizer ideas that are perfect for renal-friendly eating.

Hummus and Veggie Sticks

Hummus is a versatile and flavorful dip made from chickpeas, tahini, olive oil, lemon juice, and garlic. It's packed with protein, fiber, and healthy fats, making it an excellent choice for renal-friendly snacking. Pairing hummus with fresh vegetable sticks adds even more nutrients and crunch, making it a satisfying and nutritious snack option.

Ingredients:

- Homemade or store-bought hummus
- Assorted vegetable sticks (such as carrots, cucumbers, bell peppers, and celery)

Instructions:

1. Wash and prepare the vegetables by slicing them into sticks or bite-sized pieces.

2. Serve the vegetable sticks alongside a bowl of hummus for dipping.

3. Enjoy the hummus and veggie sticks as a healthy and satisfying snack or appetizer.

This hummus and veggie sticks combo is not only delicious but also kidney-friendly, as it's low in sodium, potassium, and phosphorus. Plus, it's easy to customize with your favorite vegetables and dip flavors, making it a versatile option for any occasion.

Cottage Cheese with Fresh Fruit

Cottage cheese is a high-protein, low-fat dairy product that's rich in calcium and other essential nutrients. Pairing cottage cheese with fresh fruit adds natural sweetness and additional vitamins and minerals, making it a nutritious and satisfying snack or appetizer option for renal-friendly eating.

Ingredients:

- Cottage cheese (low-fat or fat-free)
- Fresh fruit of your choice (such as berries, melon, pineapple, or kiwi)

Instructions:

1. Wash and prepare the fresh fruit by slicing or chopping it into bite-sized pieces.

2. Spoon the cottage cheese into a bowl or serving dish.

3. Top the cottage cheese with the fresh fruit.

4. Enjoy the cottage cheese and fresh fruit as a quick and easy snack or appetizer.

This cottage cheese and fresh fruit combo is not only delicious but also kidney-friendly, as it's low in sodium, potassium, and phosphorus. Plus, it's highly customizable, so you can mix and match your favorite fruits to suit your taste preferences and dietary needs.

Baked Sweet Potato Chips

Sweet potatoes are a nutrient-rich root vegetable that's packed with vitamins, minerals, and fiber. Baking them into crispy chips is a healthy and delicious way to enjoy them as a snack or appetizer. These homemade sweet potato chips are seasoned with herbs and spices for added flavor, making them a tasty and kidney-friendly option.

Ingredients:

- Sweet potatoes
- Olive oil

- Salt-free seasoning blend (such as garlic powder, paprika, and black pepper)

Instructions:

1. Preheat your oven to 375°F (190°C) and line a baking sheet with parchment paper.

2. Wash and peel the sweet potatoes, then slice them into thin rounds using a sharp knife or mandoline slicer.

3. In a large mixing bowl, toss the sweet potato slices with olive oil and salt-free seasoning blend until evenly coated.

4. Arrange the seasoned sweet potato slices in a single layer on the prepared baking sheet, making sure they're not overlapping.

5. Bake the sweet potato chips in the preheated oven for 15-20 minutes, flipping them halfway through, until they are golden brown and crispy.

6. Remove the sweet potato chips from the oven and let them cool slightly before serving.

7. Enjoy the baked sweet potato chips as a crunchy and flavorful snack or appetizer.

These homemade baked sweet potato chips are a healthier alternative to store-bought potato chips and are perfect for renal-friendly eating. They're low in sodium, potassium, and phosphorus, making them a nutritious and satisfying option for satisfying your snack cravings. Plus, you can customize the seasoning to suit your taste preferences, making them a versatile and delicious snack for any occasion.

CHAPTER SIX

Desserts without Compromising Kidney Health

Indulging in desserts doesn't have to mean sacrificing your kidney health. With mindful ingredient choices and creative recipes, you can enjoy delicious sweets that are both satisfying and kidney-friendly. Here are three dessert ideas that are sure to satisfy your sweet tooth without compromising kidney health.

Berry Parfait with Greek Yogurt

Greek yogurt is a protein-rich dairy product that's low in potassium and phosphorus, making it an excellent choice for individuals with kidney disease. Paired with fresh berries, which are naturally low in potassium and high in fiber and antioxidants, this berry parfait is a nutritious and delicious dessert option.

Ingredients:

- Plain Greek yogurt (low-fat or fat-free)
- Fresh berries (such as strawberries, blueberries, raspberries, or blackberries)
- Granola (low-sodium if possible)
- Honey or maple syrup (optional)

Instructions:

1. Wash and prepare the fresh berries by rinsing them under cold water and slicing any larger berries into bite-sized pieces.

2. In a glass or serving dish, layer the Greek yogurt, fresh berries, and granola, repeating until the dish is filled.

3. Drizzle a small amount of honey or maple syrup over the top if desired for added sweetness.

4. Serve the berry parfait immediately, or refrigerate it for a few hours to allow the flavors to meld together before serving.

This berry parfait with Greek yogurt is not only delicious but also kidney-friendly, as it's low in potassium and phosphorus. Plus, it's highly customizable, so you can mix and match your favorite berries and toppings to suit your taste preferences and dietary needs.

Mango Sorbet

Sorbet is a refreshing and naturally sweet dessert option that's perfect for cooling down on a hot day. This mango sorbet is made with just a few simple ingredients and is naturally low in potassium and phosphorus, making it a kidney-friendly treat.

Ingredients:

- Ripe mangoes, peeled and diced

- Fresh lime juice
- Honey or agave syrup (optional)
- Water

Instructions:

1. Place the diced mangoes in a blender or food processor and add the fresh lime juice.

2. Blend the mangoes until smooth, adding water as needed to achieve the desired consistency.

3. Taste the mango puree and add honey or agave syrup if desired for added sweetness, blending again to combine.

4. Transfer the mango puree to a shallow dish or baking pan and spread it out into an even layer.

5. Place the dish in the freezer and freeze the mango puree for 2-3 hours, stirring every 30 minutes with a fork to break up any ice crystals and create a smooth sorbet texture.

6. Once the mango sorbet is frozen and firm, scoop it into serving bowls or cones and enjoy immediately.

This mango sorbet is a delicious and kidney-friendly dessert option that's bursting with tropical flavor. It's naturally sweet and refreshing, making it a perfect treat for hot summer days or anytime you're craving something sweet but want to keep your kidney health in mind.

Baked Apples with Cinnamon

Baked apples are a comforting and satisfying dessert option that's easy to make and naturally low in potassium and phosphorus. By simply baking apples with a sprinkle of cinnamon, you can create a warm and cozy dessert that's perfect for cooler weather.

Ingredients:

- Apples (such as Granny Smith or Honeycrisp)
- Ground cinnamon
- Honey or maple syrup (optional)
- Chopped nuts (such as walnuts or almonds) (optional)

Instructions:

1. Preheat your oven to 375°F (190°C) and lightly grease a baking dish with cooking spray or butter.
2. Wash and core the apples, removing the seeds and stems but leaving the skins intact.
3. Place the cored apples in the prepared baking dish and sprinkle them generously with ground cinnamon.
4. If desired, drizzle a small amount of honey or maple syrup over the top of each apple for added sweetness.

5. Bake the apples in the preheated oven for 25-30 minutes, or until they are tender and caramelized.

6. Remove the baked apples from the oven and let them cool slightly before serving.

7. If desired, sprinkle chopped nuts over the top of the baked apples for added crunch and flavor.

8. Serve the baked apples warm, either on their own or with a dollop of Greek yogurt or a scoop of low-fat vanilla ice cream for an extra-special treat.

These baked apples with cinnamon are a delicious and kidney-friendly dessert option that's perfect for satisfying your sweet tooth without compromising your kidney health. They're warm, comforting, and bursting with natural sweetness, making them a perfect treat for any occasion. Plus, they're easy to customize with your favorite toppings and flavors, so feel free to get creative and make them your own!

CHAPTER SEVEN

Beverages to Keep You Hydrated and Healthy

Staying properly hydrated is essential for overall health and well-being, especially for individuals with kidney concerns. While water is the best choice for hydration, there are plenty of other flavorful and nutritious beverages that can help keep you hydrated while supporting kidney health. Here are three refreshing options to enjoy throughout the day.

Infused Water with Cucumber and Mint

Infused water is a simple and refreshing way to add flavor to your hydration routine without adding extra calories or sugar. This cucumber and mint infused water is not only delicious but also naturally low in potassium and phosphorus, making it a kidney-friendly choice.

Ingredients:

- Cold water
- Sliced cucumber
- Fresh mint leaves

Instructions:

1. Fill a pitcher or large jar with cold water.
2. Add slices of cucumber and fresh mint leaves to the water.
3. Stir the ingredients gently to combine.
4. Refrigerate the infused water for at least an hour to allow the flavors to meld together.
5. Serve the cucumber and mint infused water over ice, if desired, and enjoy throughout the day for a refreshing and hydrating beverage.

This infused water with cucumber and mint is a delicious and kidney-friendly alternative to sugary drinks and sodas. It's light, refreshing, and perfect for staying hydrated, especially on hot summer days.

Herbal Teas without Caffeine

Herbal teas are a comforting and hydrating beverage option that can be enjoyed hot or cold. Unlike traditional teas, herbal teas are naturally caffeine-free and come in a wide variety of flavors and blends. Choosing herbal teas without caffeine ensures that you can enjoy them anytime without interfering with your sleep or overall health.

Ingredients:

- Herbal tea bags (such as chamomile, peppermint, ginger, or hibiscus)
- Hot water

Instructions:

1. Place a herbal tea bag of your choice in a mug or teapot.
2. Pour hot water over the tea bag, covering it completely.
3. Steep the tea for the recommended amount of time, usually 5-10 minutes depending on the type of tea and your desired strength.

4. Remove the tea bag and discard it.

5. If desired, sweeten the tea with a small amount of honey or agave syrup, or enjoy it as is.

Herbal teas are a hydrating and soothing beverage option that's perfect for any time of day. Whether you prefer the calming effects of chamomile, the refreshing taste of peppermint, or the spicy warmth of ginger, there's an herbal tea to suit your taste preferences and support your kidney health.

Homemade Electrolyte Drinks

Electrolyte drinks are often marketed as sports beverages, but they can also be beneficial for individuals with kidney concerns, especially those who may be at risk of electrolyte imbalances due to medications or medical conditions. Making your own electrolyte drinks at home allows you to control the ingredients and avoid added sugars and artificial additives.

Ingredients:

- Cold water
- Freshly squeezed lemon juice
- Honey or maple syrup (optional)
- Pinch of sea salt
- Pinch of baking soda

Instructions:

1. Fill a glass with cold water.

2. Add freshly squeezed lemon juice to the water, adjusting the amount to taste.

3. If desired, sweeten the electrolyte drink with a small amount of honey or maple syrup.

4. Add a pinch of sea salt and a pinch of baking soda to the water, stirring gently to combine.

5. Taste the electrolyte drink and adjust the flavors as needed, adding more lemon juice, honey, salt, or baking soda to suit your taste preferences.

6. Serve the homemade electrolyte drink over ice, if desired, and enjoy it as a refreshing and hydrating beverage.

This homemade electrolyte drink is a natural and kidney-friendly way to replenish electrolytes and stay hydrated throughout the day. It's easy to customize with your preferred flavors and sweetness levels, making it a versatile and delicious beverage option for supporting kidney health.

CHAPTER EIGHT

Renal-Friendly Meal Prep Tips and Tricks

Maintaining a renal-friendly diet requires careful planning and preparation, but with the right strategies, meal prep can be both convenient and enjoyable. Here are three tips and tricks to help you navigate renal-friendly meal prep with ease.

Batch Cooking for Convenience

Batch cooking is a meal prep strategy that involves preparing large quantities of food at once and portioning it out for future meals. This approach can save you time and energy throughout the week while ensuring that you always have kidney-friendly meals on hand.

- Choose a day of the week to dedicate to batch cooking, such as Sunday afternoon or a free evening.

- Select renal-friendly recipes that can be easily scaled up, such as soups, stews, casseroles, and grain-based salads.

- Invest in quality food storage containers that are freezer-safe and microwave-safe for storing your batch-cooked meals.

- Cook large batches of your chosen recipes and portion them out into individual containers for easy grab-and-go meals throughout the week.

- Label each container with the name of the dish and the date it was prepared to help you keep track of freshness.

- Store some portions in the refrigerator for immediate consumption and freeze the rest for longer-term storage.

By batch cooking renal-friendly meals in advance, you can simplify your weeknight dinners and ensure that you always have nutritious options available, even on busy days.

Proper Storage of Kidney-Safe Ingredients

Proper storage of kidney-safe ingredients is essential for maintaining freshness and preventing food waste. Here are some tips for storing common renal-friendly ingredients:

- Fresh fruits and vegetables: Store fresh produce in the refrigerator in the crisper drawer or in perforated plastic bags to help maintain moisture levels. Certain fruits and vegetables, such as bananas and tomatoes, can be stored at room temperature.

- Grains and legumes: Store dried grains and legumes in airtight containers in a cool, dry pantry or cupboard. Cooked grains and legumes can be stored in the refrigerator for up to one week or frozen for longer-term storage.

- Protein sources: Store raw meat, poultry, and seafood in the refrigerator in its original packaging or in airtight containers on the bottom shelf to prevent cross-contamination. Cooked protein sources should be stored in the refrigerator for up to three days or frozen for longer-term storage.

By properly storing kidney-safe ingredients, you can prolong their shelf life and ensure that they remain fresh and safe to eat.

Planning Balanced Meals in Advance

Planning balanced meals in advance is key to maintaining a renal-friendly diet. By taking the time to plan your meals for the week ahead, you can ensure that you're getting a variety of nutrients while staying within your dietary restrictions.

- Use a meal planning template or app to map out your meals for the week, including breakfast, lunch, dinner, and snacks.

- Incorporate a balance of lean protein sources, whole grains, fresh fruits and vegetables, and healthy fats into each meal.

- Choose renal-friendly recipes that align with your dietary restrictions and taste preferences, and make a grocery list of the ingredients you'll need.

- Take inventory of your pantry, refrigerator, and freezer before heading to the grocery store to avoid buying duplicate items.

- Set aside time each week for meal prep, such as washing and chopping vegetables, cooking grains and proteins, and portioning out snacks.

- Pack your meals and snacks in reusable containers for easy transport to work, school, or other activities.

By planning balanced meals in advance, you can save time and money, reduce food waste, and ensure that you're meeting your nutritional needs while following a renal-friendly diet.

Meal prep doesn't have to be daunting, especially when you have a plan in place. By incorporating batch cooking, proper ingredient storage, and meal planning into your routine, you can streamline your renal-friendly meal prep process and set yourself up for success in maintaining a healthy diet.

CHAPTER NINE

Dining Out and Managing the Renal Diet

Eating out can be a challenge when you're following a renal diet, but with the right approach, you can still enjoy delicious meals while keeping your kidneys healthy. Here are some tips for navigating restaurant menus, making special requests, and identifying hidden sodium and potassium.

How to Navigate Restaurant Menus

When dining out on a renal diet, it's important to carefully review the menu and choose options that align with your dietary restrictions. Here's how to navigate restaurant menus effectively:

- Start by scanning the menu for renal-friendly options, such as grilled or baked proteins (chicken, fish, lean beef), steamed vegetables, and whole grains.

- Look for dishes that can be customized to meet your dietary needs, such as asking for sauces and dressings on the side or substituting high-potassium sides like French fries with lower-potassium options like steamed rice or baked potatoes.

- Pay attention to portion sizes, as restaurant servings are often larger than what you would eat at home. Consider sharing an entree with a dining companion or asking for a togo box to portion out half of your meal before you start eating.

- Be cautious of menu items that are high in sodium, such as soups, sauces, and processed meats. Opt for dishes with minimal added salt or ask if the restaurant offers low-sodium alternatives.

- Don't be afraid to ask your server questions about how dishes are prepared and whether they can accommodate special dietary needs. Most restaurants are willing to accommodate requests and make substitutions to accommodate dietary restrictions.

By carefully reviewing restaurant menus and making informed choices, you can enjoy dining out while still following your renal diet.

Tips for Making Special Requests

Making special requests when dining out can help ensure that your meal meets your dietary needs. Here are some tips for communicating your needs effectively to restaurant staff:

- Be polite and respectful when making special requests. Most restaurants are willing to accommodate dietary restrictions, but it's important to communicate your needs clearly and politely.

- Specify any dietary restrictions or allergies upfront when ordering. This will help the restaurant staff understand your needs and make appropriate accommodations.

- Be specific about your requests, such as asking for sauces and dressings on the side, requesting grilled instead of fried proteins, or substituting high-potassium sides with lower-potassium options.

- If you're unsure whether a dish meets your dietary needs, don't hesitate to ask your server for more information. They can check with the kitchen staff or provide recommendations for renal-friendly options.

- Express your appreciation to the restaurant staff for accommodating your requests. A simple thank you goes a long way and helps build positive relationships with the restaurant staff.

By making clear and specific requests, you can ensure that your meal meets your dietary needs while dining out.

Identifying Hidden Sodium and Potassium

Hidden sodium and potassium are common in restaurant dishes, so it's important to be mindful of where these ingredients may be hiding. Here are some tips for identifying hidden sodium and potassium in restaurant meals:

- Be wary of menu items that are prepared with sauces, dressings, or marinades, as these can be sources of hidden sodium and potassium. Ask for these items on the side so you can control the amount you consume.

- Watch out for processed meats, such as bacon, sausage, and deli meats, which are often high in sodium and potassium. Opt for lean proteins like grilled chicken or fish instead.

- Choose fresh or steamed vegetables over canned or pickled varieties, which may be higher in sodium. Ask if the restaurant offers fresh vegetable sides or if they can prepare vegetables without added salt.

- Avoid dishes that are heavily seasoned or fried, as these cooking methods can increase the sodium and potassium content of the dish. Look for simple, minimally seasoned options instead.

By being aware of where hidden sodium and potassium may lurk in restaurant meals, you can make informed choices that support your renal health.

Dining out on a renal diet can be challenging, but with careful planning and communication, you can enjoy delicious meals while keeping your kidneys healthy. By navigating restaurant menus thoughtfully, making special requests when needed, and being mindful of hidden sodium and potassium, you can dine out with confidence while following your renal diet.

CHAPTER TEN

Staying Motivated and Adapting to the Renal Diet

Following a renal diet can be challenging, but with the right mindset and strategies, you can stay motivated and adapt to your new way of eating. Here are some tips for staying motivated and adapting to the renal diet.

Setting Realistic Goals

Setting realistic goals is essential for staying motivated and making progress on the renal diet. Here are some tips for setting and achieving your goals:

- Start by setting small, achievable goals that are specific, measurable, and realistic. For example, aim to incorporate one new renal-friendly recipe into your meal plan each week or to reduce your sodium intake by a certain amount.

- Break larger goals down into smaller, manageable steps to make them less overwhelming. Focus on making gradual changes over time rather than trying to overhaul your entire diet all at once.

- Track your progress regularly and celebrate your achievements along the way. Keep a food journal to monitor your dietary intake and record any changes in your health or energy levels.

- Be flexible and willing to adjust your goals as needed. If you encounter setbacks or obstacles, don't be discouraged—instead, reassess your goals and make any necessary adjustments to stay on track.

By setting realistic goals and taking small, consistent steps towards achieving them, you can stay motivated and make steady progress on the renal diet.

Celebrating Small Victories

Celebrating small victories is important for staying motivated and maintaining a positive attitude on the renal diet. Here are some ideas for celebrating your achievements:

- Acknowledge and celebrate your progress, no matter how small. Whether you successfully prepared a renal-friendly meal for the first time or resisted the temptation to indulge in a high-sodium snack, take a moment to acknowledge your accomplishment and pat yourself on the back.

- Reward yourself for reaching milestones and achieving your goals. Treat yourself to something special, such as a relaxing bath, a new book, or a day out with friends, as a way to celebrate your hard work and dedication.

- Share your successes with others and celebrate together. Whether you post about your achievements on social media, share them with a supportive friend or family member, or celebrate with your renal support group, sharing your victories with others can help reinforce your motivation and inspire others to stay on track.

By celebrating small victories and recognizing your progress, you can stay motivated and maintain a positive mindset on the renal diet.

Finding Support and Resources

Finding support and resources is essential for staying motivated and adapting to the renal diet. Here are some ways to find support and access helpful resources:

- Join a renal support group or online community to connect with others who are also following the renal diet. Share your experiences, ask questions, and offer support and encouragement to others who are on a similar journey.

- Seek out reputable sources of information and educational materials on the renal diet. Look for books, websites, and online forums that provide accurate and up-to-date information about kidney health and nutrition.

- Consider working with a registered dietitian or nutritionist who specializes in kidney health. A dietitian can provide personalized guidance and support to help you navigate the renal diet and make informed dietary choices.

- Talk to your healthcare provider about any challenges or concerns you may have related to the renal diet. Your healthcare team can offer guidance, answer questions, and provide additional resources to support your journey.

By finding support and accessing helpful resources, you can stay motivated and empowered to adapt to the renal diet and prioritize your kidney health.

In conclusion, staying motivated and adapting to the renal diet requires setting realistic goals, celebrating small victories, and finding support and resources. By taking proactive steps to stay motivated and seek out support, you can successfully navigate the renal diet and maintain your kidney health for the long term.

CHAPTER ELEVEN
RENAL DIETS AND THEIR PREPARATION

Low Sodium Diet

Ingredients:

1. Fresh vegetables (e.g., spinach, kale, bell peppers, carrots)
2. Lean protein (e.g., chicken breast, fish fillets, tofu)
3. Low-sodium broth or stock
4. Whole grains (e.g., brown rice, quinoa, whole wheat pasta)
5. Fresh herbs and spices (e.g., garlic, basil, parsley)
6. Olive oil or unsaturated fats for cooking

Instructions:

1. **Preparation (5 minutes):**
   - Wash and chop vegetables.
   - Cut protein into desired portions.
   - Measure out grains according to serving size.

2. **Cooking (20 minutes):**
   - Heat a non-stick pan over medium heat.
   - Add a small amount of olive oil to the pan.

- Sauté vegetables until tender-crisp.
- In a separate pan, cook protein until fully cooked.
- Cook grains according to package instructions, using low-sodium broth or water for extra flavor.

3. **Seasoning (5 minutes):**
    - Season vegetables, protein, and grains with fresh herbs and spices. Avoid using salt or salty seasonings.
    - Taste and adjust seasoning as needed.

4. **Serving (1 minute):**
    - Plate the cooked vegetables, protein, and grains.
    - Serve immediately.

DASH Diet

Ingredients:

1. Fresh fruits (e.g., apples, bananas, berries)
2. Fresh vegetables (e.g., leafy greens, broccoli, tomatoes)
3. Lean protein (e.g., chicken breast, turkey, beans)
4. Low-fat or fat-free dairy products (e.g., milk, yogurt, cheese)
5. Whole grains (e.g., oats, whole wheat bread, brown rice)
6. Nuts and seeds (e.g., almonds, chia seeds, flaxseeds)

7. Olive oil or other unsaturated fats for cooking

Instructions:

1. **Preparation (5 minutes):**
   - Wash and chop fruits and vegetables.
   - Measure out grains and other ingredients.

2. **Cooking (20 minutes):**
   - Heat a non-stick pan over medium heat.
   - Cook protein until fully cooked, using minimal oil.
   - Steam or sauté vegetables until tender.
   - Cook grains according to package instructions, using water or low-sodium broth.
   - Prepare any additional sides, such as salads or fruit bowls.

3. **Assembling (5 minutes):**
   - Arrange cooked protein, vegetables, and grains on plates.
   - Serve with a side of low-fat or fat-free dairy, if desired.
   - Sprinkle nuts and seeds on salads or yogurt for added crunch and nutrition.

4. **Serving (1 minute):**
    - Serve immediately and enjoy your DASH-friendly meal!

Mediterranean Diet

Ingredients:

1. Fresh vegetables (e.g., tomatoes, cucumbers, bell peppers)
2. Leafy greens (e.g., spinach, kale)
3. Whole grains (e.g., couscous, bulgur, whole grain bread)
4. Lean protein (e.g., grilled chicken breast, fish fillets)
5. Healthy fats (e.g., olive oil, olives, nuts)
6. Fresh herbs and spices (e.g., basil, oregano, garlic)
7. Optional: Feta cheese, low-fat yogurt

Instructions:

1. **Preparation (5 minutes):**
    - Wash and chop vegetables and leafy greens.
    - Measure out grains and protein.
    - Prepare any additional ingredients like olives or cheese.
2. **Cooking (20 minutes):**
    - Heat a non-stick pan over medium heat.

- Cook protein (chicken or fish) until fully cooked and lightly seasoned with herbs.
- Meanwhile, prepare grains according to package instructions, using water or low-sodium broth for extra flavor.
- In a separate pan, sauté vegetables in olive oil until tender-crisp.

3. **Assembly (5 minutes):**

- Plate the cooked protein, grains, and vegetables.
- Drizzle with a little extra olive oil.
- Optionally, crumble some feta cheese on top for added flavor.

4. **Serving (1 minute):**

- Serve immediately and enjoy your Mediterranean-inspired meal!

Plant-Based Diet

Ingredients:

1. Assorted vegetables (e.g., broccoli, cauliflower, bell peppers)
2. Leafy greens (e.g., spinach, kale)
3. Legumes (e.g., chickpeas, lentils, black beans)

4. Whole grains (e.g., quinoa, brown rice, barley)

5. Nuts and seeds (e.g., almonds, pumpkin seeds, chia seeds)

6. Fresh herbs and spices (e.g., cilantro, cumin, turmeric)

7. Olive oil or other healthy fats for cooking

Instructions:

1. **Preparation (5 minutes):**
   - Wash and chop vegetables and leafy greens.
   - Rinse legumes if using canned.
   - Measure out grains and any additional ingredients.

2. **Cooking (20 minutes):**
   - Heat a non-stick pan over medium heat.
   - Sauté vegetables and leafy greens in olive oil until tender.
   - Cook grains according to package instructions, using water or low-sodium broth.
   - If using canned legumes, heat them through in a small pot or microwave.

3. **Combining (5 minutes):**

- Mix cooked grains, vegetables, and legumes together in a large bowl.
- Add nuts and seeds for extra crunch and nutrition.
- Season with herbs and spices to taste.

4. **Serving (1 minute):**
   - Serve immediately and enjoy your nutritious plant-based meal!

Low Protein Diet

Ingredients:

1. Low-protein vegetables (e.g., zucchini, eggplant, mushrooms)
2. Low-protein fruits (e.g., berries, apples, pears)
3. Grains low in protein (e.g., white rice, white pasta, corn tortillas)
4. Limited protein sources (e.g., egg whites, tofu, small amounts of chicken or fish)
5. Low-protein dairy alternatives (e.g., almond milk, rice milk)
6. Healthy fats (e.g., avocado, olive oil, nuts)

Instructions:

1. **Preparation (5 minutes):**

- Wash and chop low-protein vegetables and fruits.
- Measure out grains and limited protein sources.

2. **Cooking (20 minutes):**

    - Heat a non-stick pan over medium heat.
    - Cook limited protein sources (such as tofu or egg whites) until lightly browned.
    - Steam or sauté low-protein vegetables until tender.
    - Cook grains according to package instructions.

3. **Assembly (5 minutes):**

    - Plate the cooked limited protein sources, vegetables, and grains.
    - Add a side of low-protein fruit or a small serving of a low-protein dairy alternative.
    - Drizzle with a little olive oil for added flavor.

4. **Serving (1 minute):**

    - Serve immediately and enjoy your low-protein meal!

Ketogenic Diet

Ingredients:

1. High-fat protein sources (e.g., fatty fish, bacon, eggs)

2. Low-carb vegetables (e.g., spinach, kale, broccoli)

3. Healthy fats (e.g., avocado, olive oil, coconut oil)

4. Nuts and seeds (e.g., almonds, walnuts, chia seeds)

5. Low-carb dairy products (e.g., hard cheeses, full-fat yogurt)

6. Herbs and spices for flavoring (e.g., garlic, basil, chili powder)

Instructions:

1. **Preparation (5 minutes):**
   - Wash and chop low-carb vegetables.
   - Measure out high-fat protein sources and any additional ingredients.

2. **Cooking (20 minutes):**
   - Heat a non-stick pan over medium heat.
   - Cook high-fat protein sources until fully cooked.
   - Sauté or steam low-carb vegetables in olive oil or coconut oil.
   - Prepare any additional sides, such as a small salad with nuts and seeds.

3. **Assembly (5 minutes):**
   - Plate the cooked protein and vegetables.

- Add a side of low-carb dairy, if desired.
- Sprinkle with herbs and spices for extra flavor.

4. **Serving (1 minute):**
   - Serve immediately and enjoy your ketogenic meal!

Vegetarian Diet

Ingredients:

1. Assorted vegetables (e.g., spinach, broccoli, bell peppers)
2. Leafy greens (e.g., kale, Swiss chard)
3. Legumes (e.g., lentils, chickpeas, black beans)
4. Whole grains (e.g., quinoa, brown rice, whole wheat couscous)
5. Eggs or dairy (optional for lacto-vegetarian; choose low-protein options)
6. Nuts and seeds (e.g., almonds, sunflower seeds, chia seeds)
7. Olive oil or other healthy fats for cooking

Instructions:

1. **Preparation (5 minutes):**
   - Wash and chop vegetables and leafy greens.
   - Rinse legumes if using canned.

- Measure out grains and any additional ingredients.

2. **Cooking (20 minutes):**

    - Heat a non-stick pan over medium heat.

    - Sauté vegetables and leafy greens in olive oil until tender.

    - Cook grains according to package instructions.

    - If using canned legumes, heat them through in a small pot or microwave.

3. **Combining (5 minutes):**

    - Mix cooked grains, vegetables, and legumes together in a large bowl.

    - Optionally, add eggs or dairy if desired.

    - Top with nuts and seeds for extra texture and nutrition.

4. **Serving (1 minute):**

    - Serve immediately and enjoy your vegetarian meal!

Vegan Diet

Ingredients:

1. Assorted vegetables (e.g., broccoli, cauliflower, carrots)

2. Leafy greens (e.g., spinach, kale)

3. Legumes (e.g., lentils, chickpeas, black beans)

4. Whole grains (e.g., quinoa, brown rice, whole wheat pasta)

5. Nuts and seeds (e.g., almonds, flaxseeds, hemp seeds)

6. Olive oil or other plant-based fats for cooking

7. Plant-based milk alternatives (e.g., almond milk, oat milk)

Instructions:

1. **Preparation (5 minutes):**
    - Wash and chop vegetables and leafy greens.
    - Rinse legumes if using canned.
    - Measure out grains and any additional ingredients.

2. **Cooking (20 minutes):**
    - Heat a non-stick pan over medium heat.
    - Sauté vegetables and leafy greens in olive oil until tender.
    - Cook grains according to package instructions.
    - If using canned legumes, heat them through in a small pot or microwave.

3. **Combining (5 minutes):**

- Mix cooked grains, vegetables, and legumes together in a large bowl.
- Top with nuts and seeds for extra texture and nutrition.
- Use plant-based milk alternatives to create creamy sauces or dressings if desired.

4. **Serving (1 minute):**
   - Serve immediately and enjoy your vegan meal!

Paleo Diet

Ingredients:

1. Lean protein sources (e.g., chicken breast, turkey, lean cuts of beef or pork)
2. Fish and seafood (e.g., salmon, tuna, shrimp)
3. Fresh vegetables (e.g., broccoli, cauliflower, bell peppers)
4. Berries and other low-sugar fruits (e.g., blueberries, strawberries)
5. Nuts and seeds (e.g., almonds, walnuts, chia seeds)
6. Healthy fats (e.g., avocado, olive oil, coconut oil)

Instructions:

1. **Preparation (5 minutes):**

- Wash and chop vegetables.
- Measure out protein sources and any additional ingredients.

2. **Cooking (20 minutes):**

    - Heat a non-stick pan over medium heat.
    - Cook protein sources until fully cooked, using minimal oil.
    - Steam or sauté vegetables in olive oil or coconut oil until tender.
    - Optionally, grill or bake fish or seafood.

3. **Assembly (5 minutes):**

    - Plate the cooked protein and vegetables.
    - Serve with a side of fresh berries or a small handful of nuts and seeds.
    - Drizzle with a little olive oil or top with sliced avocado for added flavor and healthy fats.

4. **Serving (1 minute):**

    - Serve immediately and enjoy your paleo-friendly meal!

Flexitarian Diet

Ingredients:

1. Assorted vegetables (e.g., spinach, kale, bell peppers)
2. Legumes (e.g., chickpeas, black beans, lentils)
3. Whole grains (e.g., quinoa, brown rice, whole grain bread)
4. Lean protein sources (e.g., tofu, tempeh, seitan)
5. Fish and seafood (optional)
6. Eggs (optional)
7. Nuts and seeds (e.g., almonds, pumpkin seeds, flaxseeds)
8. Olive oil or other healthy fats for cooking

Instructions:

1. **Preparation (5 minutes):**
    - Wash and chop vegetables.
    - Rinse legumes if using canned.
    - Measure out grains, protein sources, and any additional ingredients.

2. **Cooking (20 minutes):**
    - Heat a non-stick pan over medium heat.
    - Cook protein sources (such as tofu or tempeh) until lightly browned.
    - Sauté vegetables in olive oil until tender.

- Cook grains according to package instructions.
- Optionally, prepare fish or seafood separately.

3. **Combining (5 minutes):**
   - Mix cooked grains, vegetables, legumes, and protein sources together in a large bowl.
   - Top with nuts and seeds for extra crunch and nutrition.
   - If desired, serve with a side of fish or seafood.

4. **Serving (1 minute):**
   - Serve immediately and enjoy your flexitarian meal!

Weight Watchers Diet

Ingredients:

1. Lean protein sources (e.g., chicken breast, turkey, fish)
2. Assorted vegetables (e.g., spinach, broccoli, carrots)
3. Fresh fruits (e.g., apples, berries, oranges)
4. Whole grains (e.g., brown rice, quinoa, whole wheat bread)
5. Low-fat dairy products (e.g., skim milk, low-fat yogurt, cottage cheese)
6. Healthy fats (e.g., avocado, olive oil, nuts)
7. Herbs and spices for flavoring (e.g., garlic, basil, cinnamon)

Instructions:

1. **Preparation (5 minutes):**
   - Wash and chop vegetables and fruits.
   - Measure out protein sources, grains, and any additional ingredients.

2. **Cooking (20 minutes):**
   - Heat a non-stick pan over medium heat.
   - Cook lean protein sources until fully cooked, using minimal oil.
   - Steam or sauté vegetables in olive oil until tender.
   - Cook grains according to package instructions.

3. **Combining (5 minutes):**
   - Mix cooked protein, vegetables, and grains together in a large bowl.
   - Serve with a side of fresh fruit.
   - Optionally, add a serving of low-fat dairy for extra protein and calcium.

4. **Serving (1 minute):**
   - Serve immediately and enjoy your Weight Watchers-friendly meal!

Atkins Diet

Ingredients:

1. Protein sources (e.g., beef, pork, chicken, fish, eggs)
2. Low-carb vegetables (e.g., spinach, broccoli, cauliflower)
3. Healthy fats (e.g., avocado, olive oil, butter)
4. Full-fat dairy products (e.g., cheese, cream, butter)
5. Nuts and seeds (e.g., almonds, macadamia nuts, chia seeds)
6. Herbs and spices for flavoring (e.g., garlic, pepper, basil)

Instructions:

1. **Preparation (5 minutes):**
   - Wash and chop low-carb vegetables.
   - Measure out protein sources, fats, and any additional ingredients.

2. **Cooking (20 minutes):**
   - Heat a non-stick pan over medium heat.
   - Cook protein sources until fully cooked, using butter or olive oil for added fat.
   - Sauté or steam low-carb vegetables in butter or olive oil until tender.

- Optionally, prepare a side salad with leafy greens and nuts/seeds.

3. **Assembly (5 minutes):**

    - Plate the cooked protein and vegetables.

    - Add a serving of full-fat dairy, such as cheese, if desired.

    - Sprinkle with herbs and spices for extra flavor.

4. **Serving (1 minute):**

    - Serve immediately and enjoy your Atkins-friendly meal!

Zone Diet

Ingredients:

1. Lean protein sources (e.g., chicken breast, turkey, fish)

2. Low-glycemic index carbohydrates (e.g., quinoa, brown rice, sweet potatoes)

3. Healthy fats (e.g., avocado, olive oil, nuts)

4. Assorted vegetables (e.g., spinach, broccoli, bell peppers)

5. Fresh fruits (e.g., berries, apples, oranges)

6. Herbs and spices for flavoring (e.g., garlic, basil, cumin)

Instructions:

1. **Preparation (5 minutes):**

- Wash and chop vegetables and fruits.
- Measure out protein sources, carbohydrates, and any additional ingredients.

2. **Cooking (20 minutes):**
   - Heat a non-stick pan over medium heat.
   - Cook lean protein sources until fully cooked, using minimal oil.
   - Steam or sauté vegetables in olive oil until tender.
   - Cook carbohydrates according to package instructions.

3. **Combining (5 minutes):**
   - Divide the cooked protein, carbohydrates, and vegetables into balanced portions.
   - Add a serving of fresh fruit to each portion.
   - Drizzle with a little olive oil or sprinkle with herbs and spices for extra flavor.

4. **Serving (1 minute):**
   - Serve immediately and enjoy your Zone Diet-friendly meal!

Whole30 Diet

Ingredients:

1. Whole foods including:

    - Lean protein sources (e.g., chicken breast, turkey, fish)
    - Assorted vegetables (e.g., spinach, broccoli, cauliflower)
    - Fresh fruits (e.g., berries, apples, oranges)
    - Healthy fats (e.g., avocado, olive oil, coconut oil)
    - Nuts and seeds (e.g., almonds, cashews, chia seeds)

2. Herbs and spices for flavoring (e.g., garlic, basil, paprika)

Instructions:

1. **Preparation (5 minutes):**

    - Wash and chop vegetables and fruits.
    - Measure out protein sources, fats, and any additional ingredients.

2. **Cooking (20 minutes):**

    - Heat a non-stick pan over medium heat.
    - Cook lean protein sources until fully cooked, using minimal oil.
    - Steam or sauté vegetables in olive oil or coconut oil until tender.

- Optionally, toast nuts and seeds in a dry pan for added flavor and crunch.

3. **Assembly (5 minutes):**
    - Plate the cooked protein and vegetables.
    - Serve with a side of fresh fruit.
    - Optionally, sprinkle nuts and seeds over the meal for added texture and nutrition.

4. **Serving (1 minute):**
    - Serve immediately and enjoy your Whole30 Diet-friendly meal!

Renal Diabetic Diet

Ingredients:

1. Lean protein sources (e.g., chicken breast, turkey, fish)
2. Low-glycemic index carbohydrates (e.g., quinoa, brown rice, whole grain bread)
3. Non-starchy vegetables (e.g., spinach, broccoli, cauliflower)
4. Fresh fruits (e.g., berries, apples, oranges)
5. Healthy fats (e.g., avocado, olive oil, nuts)
6. Herbs and spices for flavoring (e.g., garlic, basil, cinnamon)

Instructions:

1. **Preparation (5 minutes):**

    - Wash and chop vegetables and fruits.

    - Measure out protein sources, carbohydrates, and any additional ingredients.

2. **Cooking (20 minutes):**

    - Heat a non-stick pan over medium heat.

    - Cook lean protein sources until fully cooked, using minimal oil.

    - Steam or sauté non-starchy vegetables in olive oil until tender.

    - Cook carbohydrates according to package instructions.

3. **Combining (5 minutes):**

    - Divide the cooked protein, carbohydrates, and vegetables into balanced portions.

    - Add a serving of fresh fruit to each portion.

    - Drizzle with a little olive oil or sprinkle with herbs and spices for extra flavor.

4. **Serving (1 minute):**

- Serve immediately and enjoy your Renal Diabetic Diet-friendly meal!

Renal Stone Diet

Ingredients:

1. Plenty of water
2. Low-oxalate vegetables (e.g., kale, collard greens, bell peppers)
3. Low-oxalate fruits (e.g., apples, pears, berries)
4. Lean protein sources (e.g., chicken breast, turkey, fish)
5. Whole grains (e.g., brown rice, quinoa, whole wheat bread)
6. Healthy fats (e.g., olive oil, avocado, nuts)
7. Herbs and spices for flavoring (e.g., garlic, basil, parsley)

Instructions:

1. **Preparation (5 minutes):**
   - Wash and chop low-oxalate vegetables and fruits.
   - Measure out protein sources, whole grains, and any additional ingredients.

2. **Cooking (20 minutes):**
   - Heat a non-stick pan over medium heat.

- Cook lean protein sources until fully cooked, using minimal oil.
- Steam or sauté low-oxalate vegetables in olive oil until tender.
- Cook whole grains according to package instructions.

3. **Combining (5 minutes):**

    - Combine cooked protein, whole grains, and vegetables in a balanced portion.
    - Serve with a side of low-oxalate fruits.
    - Drizzle with a little olive oil or sprinkle with herbs and spices for extra flavor.

4. **Serving (1 minute):**

    - Serve immediately and enjoy your Renal Stone Diet-friendly meal!

Low Phosphorus Diet

Ingredients:

1. Low-phosphorus protein sources (e.g., chicken breast, turkey, fish)
2. Low-phosphorus grains and starches (e.g., white rice, white bread, pasta)

3. Low-phosphorus fruits (e.g., apples, berries, grapes)

4. Low-phosphorus vegetables (e.g., green beans, cauliflower, bell peppers)

5. Healthy fats (e.g., olive oil, avocado, nuts)

6. Herbs and spices for flavoring (e.g., garlic, basil, parsley)

Instructions:

1. **Preparation (5 minutes):**

   - Wash and chop vegetables and fruits.
   - Measure out low-phosphorus protein sources, grains, and any additional ingredients.

2. **Cooking (20 minutes):**

   - Heat a non-stick pan over medium heat.
   - Cook low-phosphorus protein sources until fully cooked, using minimal oil.
   - Prepare low-phosphorus grains or starches according to package instructions.
   - Steam or sauté low-phosphorus vegetables in olive oil until tender.

3. **Combining (5 minutes):**

- Combine cooked protein, grains, and vegetables in a balanced portion.
- Serve with a side of low-phosphorus fruits.
- Drizzle with a little olive oil or sprinkle with herbs and spices for extra flavor.

4. **Serving (1 minute):**

- Serve immediately and enjoy your Low Phosphorus Diet-friendly meal!

Low Potassium Diet

Ingredients:

1. Low-potassium fruits (e.g., apples, berries, grapes)
2. Low-potassium vegetables (e.g., green beans, cauliflower, bell peppers)
3. Low-potassium grains and starches (e.g., white rice, white bread, pasta)
4. Low-potassium protein sources (e.g., chicken breast, turkey, fish)
5. Healthy fats (e.g., olive oil, avocado, nuts)
6. Herbs and spices for flavoring (e.g., garlic, basil, parsley)

Instructions:

1. **Preparation (5 minutes):**

    - Wash and chop vegetables and fruits.

    - Measure out low-potassium protein sources, grains, and any additional ingredients.

2. **Cooking (20 minutes):**

    - Heat a non-stick pan over medium heat.

    - Cook low-potassium protein sources until fully cooked, using minimal oil.

    - Prepare low-potassium grains or starches according to package instructions.

    - Steam or sauté low-potassium vegetables in olive oil until tender.

3. **Combining (5 minutes):**

    - Combine cooked protein, grains, and vegetables in a balanced portion.

    - Serve with a side of low-potassium fruits.

    - Drizzle with a little olive oil or sprinkle with herbs and spices for extra flavor.

4. **Serving (1 minute):**

- Serve immediately and enjoy your Low Potassium Diet-friendly meal!

Low Oxalate Diet

Ingredients:

1. Low-oxalate vegetables (e.g., kale, collard greens, bell peppers)
2. Low-oxalate fruits (e.g., apples, pears, berries)
3. Low-oxalate grains (e.g., white rice, quinoa, whole wheat bread)
4. Low-oxalate protein sources (e.g., chicken breast, turkey, fish)
5. Healthy fats (e.g., olive oil, avocado, nuts)
6. Herbs and spices for flavoring (e.g., garlic, basil, parsley)

Instructions:

1. **Preparation (5 minutes):**
    - Wash and chop low-oxalate vegetables and fruits.
    - Measure out low-oxalate grains, protein sources, and any additional ingredients.
2. **Cooking (20 minutes):**
    - Heat a non-stick pan over medium heat.

- Cook low-oxalate protein sources until fully cooked, using minimal oil.
- Steam or sauté low-oxalate vegetables in olive oil until tender.
- Prepare low-oxalate grains according to package instructions.

3. **Combining (5 minutes):**

- Combine cooked protein, grains, and vegetables in a balanced portion.
- Serve with a side of low-oxalate fruits.
- Drizzle with a little olive oil or sprinkle with herbs and spices for extra flavor.

4. **Serving (1 minute):**

- Serve immediately and enjoy your Low Oxalate Diet-friendly meal!

Renal Transplant Diet

Ingredients:

1. Lean protein sources (e.g., chicken breast, turkey, fish)
2. Low-sodium vegetables (e.g., spinach, kale, bell peppers)
3. Low-phosphorus grains (e.g., white rice, quinoa, couscous)

4. Low-potassium fruits (e.g., apples, berries, grapes)

5. Healthy fats (e.g., olive oil, avocado, nuts)

6. Herbs and spices for flavoring (e.g., garlic, basil, parsley)

Instructions:

1. **Preparation (5 minutes):**

    - Wash and chop vegetables and fruits.

    - Measure out protein sources, grains, and any additional ingredients.

2. **Cooking (20 minutes):**

    - Heat a non-stick pan over medium heat.

    - Cook lean protein sources until fully cooked, using minimal oil.

    - Steam or sauté low-sodium vegetables in olive oil until tender.

    - Prepare low-phosphorus grains according to package instructions.

3. **Combining (5 minutes):**

    - Combine cooked protein, grains, and vegetables in a balanced portion.

    - Serve with a side of low-potassium fruits.

- Drizzle with a little olive oil or sprinkle with herbs and spices for extra flavor.

4. **Serving (1 minute):**
    - Serve immediately and enjoy your Renal Transplant Diet-friendly meal!

Gluten-Free Diet

Ingredients:

1. Gluten-free grains (e.g., quinoa, brown rice, gluten-free pasta)
2. Lean protein sources (e.g., chicken breast, turkey, fish)
3. Fresh vegetables (e.g., spinach, broccoli, bell peppers)
4. Fresh fruits (e.g., apples, berries, oranges)
5. Healthy fats (e.g., avocado, olive oil, nuts)
6. Herbs and spices for flavoring (e.g., garlic, basil, turmeric)

Instructions:

1. **Preparation (5 minutes):**
    - Wash and chop vegetables and fruits.
    - Measure out gluten-free grains and protein sources.

2. **Cooking (20 minutes):**

- Heat a non-stick pan over medium heat.
- Cook lean protein sources until fully cooked, using minimal oil.
- Steam or sauté fresh vegetables in olive oil until tender.
- Prepare gluten-free grains according to package instructions.

3. **Combining (5 minutes):**

    - Combine cooked protein, grains, and vegetables in a balanced portion.
    - Serve with a side of fresh fruit.
    - Drizzle with a little olive oil or sprinkle with herbs and spices for extra flavor.

4. **Serving (1 minute):**

    - Serve immediately and enjoy your Gluten-Free Diet-friendly meal!

Anti-Inflammatory Diet

Ingredients:

1. Omega-3 fatty acids sources (e.g., salmon, walnuts, flaxseeds)
2. Fresh fruits (e.g., berries, oranges, pineapple)

3. Fresh vegetables (e.g., leafy greens, broccoli, tomatoes)

4. Lean protein sources (e.g., chicken breast, tofu, lentils)

5. Whole grains (e.g., quinoa, brown rice, whole wheat bread)

6. Herbs and spices with anti-inflammatory properties (e.g., turmeric, ginger, garlic)

7. Healthy fats (e.g., olive oil, avocado, nuts)

Instructions:

1. **Preparation (5 minutes):**
   - Wash and chop vegetables and fruits.
   - Measure out protein sources and whole grains.

2. **Cooking (20 minutes):**
   - Heat a non-stick pan over medium heat.
   - Cook lean protein sources until fully cooked, using minimal oil.
   - Steam or sauté fresh vegetables in olive oil until tender.
   - Prepare whole grains according to package instructions.

3. **Combining (5 minutes):**
   - Combine cooked protein, grains, and vegetables in a balanced portion.

- Serve with a side of fresh fruit.
- Drizzle with a little olive oil and sprinkle with anti-inflammatory herbs and spices for extra flavor.

4. **Serving (1 minute):**
   - Serve immediately and enjoy your Anti-Inflammatory Diet-friendly meal!

Renal Dietitian Prescribed Diet

Ingredients:

1. Low-sodium protein sources (e.g., chicken breast, turkey, fish)
2. Low-potassium vegetables (e.g., spinach, cauliflower, bell peppers)
3. Low-phosphorus grains (e.g., white rice, quinoa, couscous)
4. Low-sugar fruits (e.g., berries, apples, oranges)
5. Healthy fats (e.g., olive oil, avocado, nuts)
6. Herbs and spices for flavoring (e.g., garlic, basil, parsley)

Instructions:

1. **Preparation (5 minutes):**
   - Wash and chop vegetables and fruits.

- Measure out protein sources, grains, and any additional ingredients as prescribed by the renal dietitian.

2. **Cooking (20 minutes):**

    - Heat a non-stick pan over medium heat.

    - Cook low-sodium protein sources until fully cooked, using minimal oil.

    - Steam or sauté low-potassium vegetables in olive oil until tender.

    - Prepare low-phosphorus grains according to package instructions.

3. **Combining (5 minutes):**

    - Combine cooked protein, grains, and vegetables in a balanced portion as prescribed by the renal dietitian.

    - Serve with a side of low-sugar fruits if permitted.

    - Drizzle with a little olive oil or sprinkle with herbs and spices for extra flavor as per dietitian's recommendations.

4. **Serving (1 minute):**

    - Serve immediately and enjoy your Renal Dietitian Prescribed Diet-friendly meal!

Carb Cycling Diet

Ingredients:

1. High-carb days:

    - Complex carbohydrates (e.g., sweet potatoes, brown rice, quinoa)
    - Lean protein sources (e.g., chicken breast, turkey, fish)
    - Low-fat dairy products (e.g., skim milk, low-fat yogurt)
    - Fresh fruits (e.g., berries, apples, oranges)
    - Vegetables (e.g., spinach, broccoli, bell peppers)
    - Healthy fats in moderation (e.g., avocado, nuts, olive oil)

2. Low-carb days:

    - Lean protein sources (e.g., chicken breast, turkey, fish)
    - Non-starchy vegetables (e.g., leafy greens, cauliflower, zucchini)
    - Healthy fats (e.g., avocado, nuts, olive oil)
    - Minimal to no complex carbohydrates or fruits

Instructions:

1. **Preparation (5 minutes):**

    - Determine whether it's a high-carb or low-carb day.

- Wash and chop vegetables and fruits accordingly.
- Measure out protein sources, grains (on high-carb days), and any additional ingredients.

2. **Cooking (20 minutes):**

   - Heat a non-stick pan over medium heat.
   - Cook protein sources until fully cooked, using minimal oil.
   - Steam or sauté vegetables in olive oil until tender.
   - Prepare complex carbohydrates if it's a high-carb day, according to package instructions.

3. **Combining (5 minutes):**

   - On high-carb days, combine cooked protein, complex carbohydrates, vegetables, and fruits in appropriate portions.
   - On low-carb days, focus on a higher protein and vegetable intake, with moderate healthy fats.
   - Adjust portion sizes and ingredients based on the specific requirements of each carb cycling day.

4. **Serving (1 minute):**

   - Serve immediately and enjoy your Carb Cycling Diet-friendly meal!

Renal Diet for Children

Ingredients:

1. Kidney-friendly protein sources (e.g., chicken breast, turkey, fish)
2. Low-potassium vegetables (e.g., green beans, cauliflower, carrots)
3. Low-phosphorus grains (e.g., white rice, pasta, couscous)
4. Low-sugar fruits (e.g., apples, berries, grapes)
5. Healthy fats (e.g., avocado, olive oil, nuts)
6. Dairy or dairy alternatives (e.g., low-fat milk, yogurt, cheese)
7. Herbs and spices for flavoring (e.g., garlic powder, basil, cinnamon)
8. Child-friendly snacks (e.g., unsalted pretzels, rice cakes, apple slices)

Instructions:

1. **Preparation (5 minutes):**
   - Wash and chop vegetables and fruits into child-friendly sizes.
   - Measure out protein sources, grains, and any additional ingredients.

2. **Cooking (20 minutes):**

    - Heat a non-stick pan over medium heat.

    - Cook kidney-friendly protein sources until fully cooked, using minimal oil.

    - Steam or sauté low-potassium vegetables until tender.

    - Prepare low-phosphorus grains according to package instructions.

3. **Combining (5 minutes):**

    - Combine cooked protein, grains, and vegetables in child-sized portions.

    - Serve with a side of low-sugar fruits or a small serving of dairy.

    - Drizzle with a little olive oil or sprinkle with child-friendly herbs and spices for extra flavor.

4. **Serving (1 minute):**

    - Serve immediately and encourage your child to enjoy their Renal Diet-friendly meal!

Low-Fat Diet

Ingredients:

1. Lean protein sources (e.g., chicken breast, turkey, fish)

2. Low-fat dairy or dairy alternatives (e.g., skim milk, low-fat yogurt, tofu)

3. Non-starchy vegetables (e.g., spinach, broccoli, bell peppers)

4. Whole grains (e.g., quinoa, brown rice, whole wheat bread)

5. Fresh fruits (e.g., berries, apples, oranges)

6. Healthy fats in moderation (e.g., avocado, olive oil, nuts)

7. Herbs and spices for flavoring (e.g., garlic, basil, paprika)

Instructions:

1. **Preparation (5 minutes):**
   - Wash and chop vegetables and fruits.
   - Measure out lean protein sources, dairy or dairy alternatives, grains, and any additional ingredients.

2. **Cooking (20 minutes):**
   - Heat a non-stick pan over medium heat.
   - Cook lean protein sources until fully cooked, using minimal oil.
   - Steam or sauté non-starchy vegetables in olive oil until tender.
   - Prepare whole grains according to package instructions.

3. **Combining (5 minutes):**

    - Combine cooked protein, grains, and vegetables in balanced portions.
    - Serve with a side of fresh fruit.
    - Use low-fat dairy or dairy alternatives to add creaminess or flavor to dishes.

4. **Serving (1 minute):**

    - Serve immediately and enjoy your Low-Fat Diet-friendly meal!

Renal Diet for Elderly

Ingredients:

1. Kidney-friendly protein sources (e.g., chicken breast, turkey, fish)
2. Low-potassium vegetables (e.g., green beans, cauliflower, carrots)
3. Low-phosphorus grains (e.g., white rice, pasta, couscous)
4. Low-sugar fruits (e.g., apples, berries, grapes)
5. Healthy fats (e.g., avocado, olive oil, nuts)
6. Dairy or dairy alternatives (e.g., low-fat milk, yogurt, cheese)

7. Herbs and spices for flavoring (e.g., garlic powder, basil, cinnamon)

8. Soft or easy-to-chew options for elderly individuals

Instructions:

1. **Preparation (5 minutes):**
   - Wash and chop vegetables and fruits into manageable sizes.
   - Prepare soft or easy-to-chew protein sources if needed.
   - Measure out grains, dairy, and any additional ingredients.

2. **Cooking (20 minutes):**
   - Heat a non-stick pan over medium heat.
   - Cook kidney-friendly protein sources until fully cooked, ensuring they are soft and easy to chew.
   - Steam or sauté low-potassium vegetables until tender.
   - Prepare low-phosphorus grains according to package instructions.

3. **Combining (5 minutes):**
   - Combine cooked protein, grains, and vegetables in balanced portions.

- Serve with a side of low-sugar fruits or a small serving of dairy.
- Use soft or easy-to-chew options for elderly individuals as needed.

4. **Serving (1 minute):**
   - Serve immediately and ensure elderly individuals can comfortably enjoy their Renal Diet-friendly meal!

Intermittent Fasting

Important Note: Intermittent fasting involves cycling between periods of eating and fasting. It's crucial to consult with a healthcare professional, especially for elderly individuals or those with specific health conditions, before starting an intermittent fasting regimen.

Ingredients:

1. High-nutrient, kidney-friendly foods to support health during eating periods
2. Plenty of water during fasting periods
3. Low-potassium, low-phosphorus, low-sugar options to break the fast
4. Soft or easy-to-chew options for elderly individuals, especially during eating windows

Instructions:

1. **Eating Period:**

   - During the eating window, focus on nutrient-dense, kidney-friendly foods such as lean protein sources, low-potassium vegetables, whole grains, and healthy fats.

   - Ensure elderly individuals have access to soft or easy-to-chew options if needed.

   - Include plenty of water to stay hydrated throughout the day.

2. **Fasting Period:**

   - Encourage elderly individuals to drink plenty of water to stay hydrated during the fasting period.

   - Avoid foods and beverages during fasting hours to adhere to the fasting regimen.

3. **Breaking the Fast:**

   - When breaking the fast, choose low-potassium, low-phosphorus, and low-sugar options to ease digestion and prevent potential issues.

   - Include soft or easy-to-chew options for elderly individuals, especially if they have any difficulty with chewing or swallowing.

4. **Serving:**

    - Serve meals and snacks in accordance with the intermittent fasting schedule, ensuring elderly individuals can comfortably adhere to the regimen.

    - Monitor their health and well-being closely, adjusting the fasting schedule or meal options as needed to ensure their nutritional needs are met.

Renal Diet for Athletes

Ingredients:

1. High-quality protein sources (e.g., chicken breast, turkey, fish, lean beef)

2. Low-potassium vegetables (e.g., green beans, cauliflower, carrots)

3. Low-phosphorus grains (e.g., white rice, pasta, quinoa)

4. High-carbohydrate options for energy (e.g., whole grains, fruits, starchy vegetables)

5. Healthy fats for sustained energy (e.g., avocado, olive oil, nuts)

6. Electrolyte-rich foods to replenish electrolytes lost through sweat (e.g., bananas, coconut water, spinach)

7. Herbs and spices for flavoring (e.g., garlic, basil, parsley)

Instructions:

1. **Preparation (5 minutes):**

    - Wash and chop vegetables.

    - Measure out protein sources, grains, fruits, and any additional ingredients.

2. **Cooking (20 minutes):**

    - Heat a non-stick pan over medium heat.

    - Cook protein sources until fully cooked, incorporating herbs and spices for flavor.

    - Steam or sauté low-potassium vegetables until tender.

    - Prepare grains according to package instructions.

3. **Combining (5 minutes):**

    - Combine cooked protein, grains, and vegetables in a balanced portion.

    - Serve with a side of carbohydrate-rich fruits or starchy vegetables for energy replenishment.

    - Incorporate healthy fats for sustained energy and satiety.

    - Hydrate with electrolyte-rich foods and beverages to replenish electrolytes lost during exercise.

4. **Serving (1 minute):**

    - Serve immediately and enjoy your Renal Diet-friendly meal, tailored to support athletic performance!

Renal Diet for Pregnancy

Ingredients:

1. High-quality protein sources (e.g., chicken breast, turkey, fish, tofu)

2. Low-potassium vegetables (e.g., spinach, cauliflower, bell peppers)

3. Low-phosphorus grains (e.g., quinoa, brown rice, whole wheat bread)

4. Calcium-rich foods for fetal development (e.g., low-fat dairy, tofu, leafy greens)

5. Iron-rich foods to prevent anemia (e.g., lean meat, beans, lentils, fortified cereals)

6. Folic acid-rich foods to prevent birth defects (e.g., leafy greens, citrus fruits, fortified grains)

7. Healthy fats for brain development (e.g., avocado, olive oil, nuts)

8. Herbs and spices for flavoring (e.g., garlic, basil, ginger)

Instructions:

1. **Preparation (5 minutes):**

    - Wash and chop vegetables.

    - Measure out protein sources, grains, dairy, fruits, and any additional ingredients.

2. **Cooking (20 minutes):**

    - Heat a non-stick pan over medium heat.

    - Cook protein sources until fully cooked, incorporating herbs and spices for flavor.

    - Steam or sauté low-potassium vegetables until tender.

    - Prepare grains according to package instructions.

3. **Combining (5 minutes):**

    - Combine cooked protein, grains, and vegetables in a balanced portion.

    - Incorporate calcium-rich foods to support fetal bone development.

    - Ensure adequate intake of iron-rich foods to prevent anemia during pregnancy.

    - Include folic acid-rich foods to support neural tube development in the fetus.

- Incorporate healthy fats for fetal brain development and maternal health.

4. **Serving (1 minute):**

    - Serve immediately and enjoy your Renal Diet-friendly meal, designed to support a healthy pregnancy!

These recipes provide quick and nutritious options for athletes and pregnant individuals following a Renal Diet, tailored to meet their specific nutritional needs during these life stages.

THE END

www.ingramcontent.com/pod-product-compliance
Lightning Source LLC
Chambersburg PA
CBHW062219220526
45471CB00009B/3271